Cholangioscopy

Shyam Menon · Venkata Lekharaju ·
Christopher Wadsworth ·
Laura Dwyer · Richard Sturgess

Cholangioscopy

A Practical Guide and Atlas

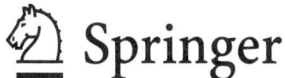

Shyam Menon
Department of Gastroenterology
New Cross Hospital
The Royal Wolverhampton
Hospitals NHS Trust
Wolverhampton, UK

Venkata Lekharaju
Department of Gastroenterology
Arrowe Park Hospital
Wirral University Teaching
Hospital NHS Foundation Trust
Wirral, UK

Christopher Wadsworth
Department of Gastroenterology
Hammersmith Hospital
Imperial College London
London, UK

Laura Dwyer
Department of Gastroenterology
Aintree University Hospitals
NHS Foundation Trust
Liverpool, UK

Richard Sturgess
Department of Gastroenterology
Aintree University Hospitals NHS
Foundation Trust
Liverpool, UK

ISBN 978-3-030-27260-9   ISBN 978-3-030-27261-6 (eBook)
https://doi.org/10.1007/978-3-030-27261-6

© Springer Nature Switzerland AG 2020

This work is subject to copyright. All rights are reserved by the Publisher, whether the whole or part of the material is concerned, specifically the rights of translation, reprinting, reuse of illustrations, recitation, broadcasting, reproduction on microfilms or in any other physical way, and transmission or information storage and retrieval, electronic adaptation, computer software, or by similar or dissimilar methodology now known or hereafter developed.

The use of general descriptive names, registered names, trademarks, service marks, etc. in this publication does not imply, even in the absence of a specific statement, that such names are exempt from the relevant protective laws and regulations and therefore free for general use.

The publisher, the authors and the editors are safe to assume that the advice and information in this book are believed to be true and accurate at the date of publication. Neither the publisher nor the authors or the editors give a warranty, expressed or implied, with respect to the material contained herein or for any errors or omissions that may have been made. The publisher remains neutral with regard to jurisdictional claims in published maps and institutional affiliations.

This Springer imprint is published by the registered company Springer Nature Switzerland AG

The registered company address is: Gewerbestrasse 11, 6330 Cham, Switzerland

Preface

The book and videos have been specifically developed to encompass the team involved in delivering cholangioscopy and we feel that it will be of value to nurses assisting in cholangioscopy and trainees, in addition to practising hepatobiliary endoscopists. The online videos are integral to the book and focus on the practical aspects of assembling and using the system, with video examples of the application of cholangioscopy in different settings.

Wolverhampton, UK	Shyam Menon
Wirral, UK	Venkata Lekharaju
London, UK	Christopher Wadsworth
Liverpool, UK	Laura Dwyer
Liverpool, UK	Richard Sturgess

particularly within the gastric fundus or the deep portion of the duodenum [13]. Hence, this technique is not as popular as compared to single operator cholangioscopy. However, the advantages of direct cholangioscopy are superior endoscopic views and a larger accessory channel within the endoscope, which can accommodate larger biopsy forceps and other accessories such as argon plasma coagulation (APC) catheters.

Hepatobiliary Anatomy

The important anatomical landmarks while performing cholangioscopy are the ampulla of vater (major papilla), common bile duct, cystic duct and common bile duct confluence, common hepatic duct, hilum and intrahepatic ducts. Intrahepatic ducts can be divided further into right anterior, right posterior and left intrahepatic ducts.

Cholangioscopic appearance of the normal ductal mucosa has a creamy/pearly colour with a well-defined vascular pattern. Villous formation is also more noticeable in the distal bile duct, adjacent to the papilla.

Ampulla

The normal ampulla (also termed the major papilla) varies considerable in size, shape and appearance and is generally seen as a circular/valvular structure on the medical wall of the second part of the duodenum. The course of the bile duct may be obvious as a longitudinal bulge into the lumen for 1–2 cm above the major papilla. A horizontal duodenal muscular fold may sometimes hide the major papilla. The orifice of the bile duct is at the apex of the papillary structure. The major papilla may be patulous with several fleshy fronds of protruding mucosa or may be obscured by duodenal folds.

Common Bile Duct

The common hepatic duct continues inferiorly into the common bile duct, with the cystic duct commonly inserting into the common hepatic duct but occasionally into the common bile duct. Anatomically, the common bile duct generally courses anterior to the portal vein. The hepatic artery is usually located slightly laterally, with the duct, artery and vein comprising the portal triad.

Cystic Duct—Common Bile Duct Confluence

This is an important anatomical landmark for difficult bile duct stones requiring cholangioscopy-guided therapy. Stones situated at the cystic duct-common bile duct junction can be challenging to extract using conventional endoscopic techniques.

The cystic duct joins the bile duct in the following ways:

1. Low insertion of the cystic duct—cystic duct joins the distal thirds of the bile duct
2. Medial insertion—cystic duct drains into the left side of the common hepatic duct
3. Parallel course—cystic duct runs parallel to common hepatic duct for at least 2 centimetres (cm).

Intrahepatic Ducts

The classic biliary anatomy appears in only 58% of the population [14]. It consists of the right and left hepatic ducts draining the right and left lobes of the liver respectively and joining at the hilum to form the common hepatic duct. The functional classification of liver segments by Couinaud [15] divides the liver into eight distinct functional segments or units (Figs. 1.1 and 1.2). The right main intrahepatic duct branches into the right

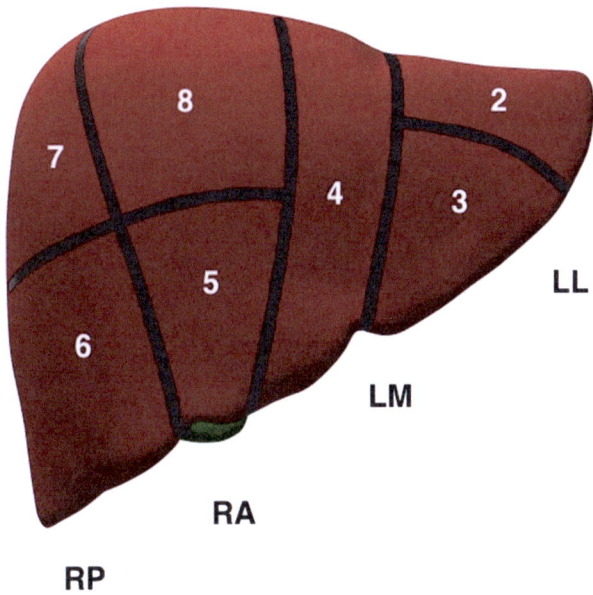

Fig. 1.1 Couinaud's classification of liver segments. In this anterior view of the liver, LL (left lateral, liver segments 2 and 3) and LM (left medial: liver segment 4) comprise the left lobe. RA (right anterior: segments 5 and 8) and RP (right posterior: segments 6 and 7) comprise the right lobe of the liver

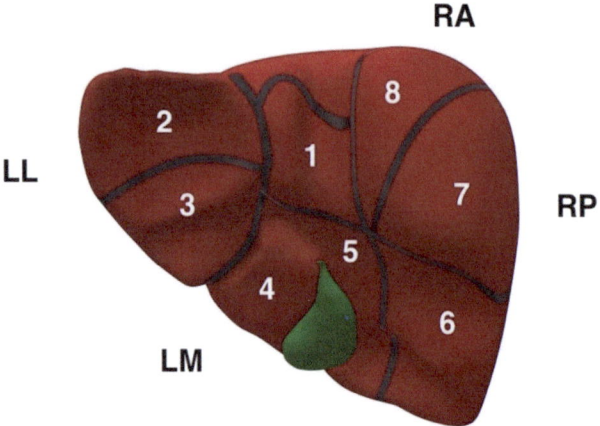

Fig. 1.2 Couinaud's classification of liver segments. In this posterior view of the liver, LL (left lateral, liver segments 2 and 3) and LM (left medial: liver segments 1 and 4) comprise the left lobe. RA (right anterior: segments 5 and 8) and RP (right posterior: segments 6 and 7) comprise the right lobe of the liver

posterior duct draining the right posterior segments (VI and VII) and the right anterior duct draining the anterior segments (V and VIII) [15] (Fig. 1.3). Segmental tributaries draining the left lateral segment (II) and the left medical segment (IV) form the left main intrahepatic duct. Anatomical variants of the biliary system are important for endoscopists to be aware of while performing cholangioscopy and advanced hepatobiliary endoscopy.

A few variants that may be observed are:

1. Right posterior duct draining into the left hepatic duct
2. Right posterior duct joining the right anterior duct
3. Triple confluence: right posterior, right anterior and left hepatic ducts joining at the same point to form the common hepatic duct
4. Right posterior duct draining into the common hepatic duct or cystic duct.

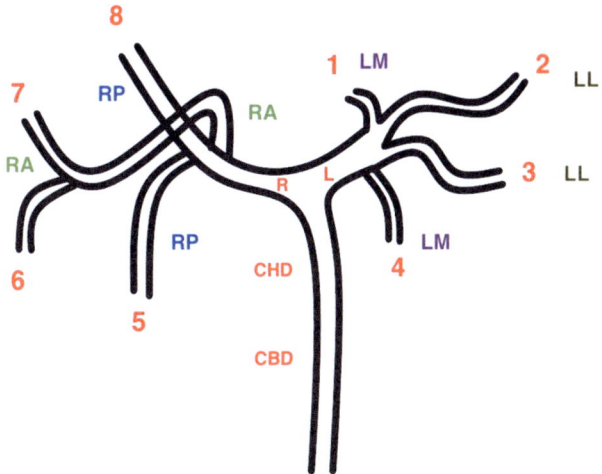

Fig. 1.3 Anatomy of the biliary system in relation to Couinaud's liver segments. The common bile duct (CBD) extends into the common hepatic duct (CHD), which then splits into the right (R) and left (L) main ducts. The right anterior (RA) and the right posterior (RP) segmental ducts take off from the right main duct to provide sectoral drainage to segments 6 and 7 (RA) and segments 5 and 8 (RP). Sectoral ducts 1 and 4 (LM: left medial) and 2 and 3 (LL: left lateral) provide drainage to the left lobe of the liver

References

1. Neuhaus H. Cholangioscopy. Endoscopy. 1992;24:125–32.
2. Ayoub F, Yang D, Draganov PV. Cholangioscopy in the digital era. Transl Gastroenterol Hepatol. 2018;3:82.
3. Bokemeyer A, et al. Digital single-operator cholangioscopy: a useful tool for selective guidewire placements across complex biliary strictures. Surg Endosc. 2018.
4. Bogardus ST, et al. "Mother-baby" biliary endoscopy: the University of Chicago experience. Am J Gastroenterol. 1996;91(1):105–10.
5. Voaklander R, et al. An overview of the evolution of direct cholangioscopy techniques for diagnosis and therapy. Gastroenterol Hepatol (N Y). 2016;12(7):433–7.

6. Nguyen NQ, Binmoeller KF, Shah JN. Cholangioscopy and pancreatoscopy (with videos). Gastrointest Endosc. 2009;70(6):1200–10.
7. Itoi T. Cholangioscopy. In: Jonnalagadda S, editor. Gastrointestinal endoscopy. New York: Springer Science + Business Media; 2015. p. 23–35.
8. Chen YK, Pleskow DK. SpyGlass single-operator peroral cholangiopancreatoscopy system for the diagnosis and therapy of bile-duct disorders: a clinical feasibility study (with video). Gastrointest Endosc. 2007;65(6):832–41.
9. Chen YK, et al. Single-operator cholangioscopy in patients requiring evaluation of bile duct disease or therapy of biliary stones (with videos). Gastrointest Endosc. 2011;74(4):805–14.
10. Draganov P. The SpyGlass(R) direct visualization system for cholangioscopy. Gastroenterol Hepatol (NY). 2008;4(7):469–70.
11. Shah RJ, et al. Randomized study of digital single-operator cholangioscope compared to fiberoptic single-operator cholangioscope in a novel cholangioscopy bench model. Endosc Int Open. 2018;6(7):E851–6.
12. Yasuda I, Itoi T. Recent advances in endoscopic management of difficult bile duct stones. Dig Endosc. 2013;25(4):376–85.
13. Larghi A, Waxman I. Endoscopic direct cholangioscopy by using an ultra-slim upper endoscope: a feasibility study. Gastrointest Endosc. 2006;63(6):853–7.
14. Catalano OA, et al. Vascular and biliary variants in the liver: implications for liver surgery. RadioGraphics. 2008;28(2):359–79.
15. Couinaud C. The paracaval segments of the liver. J Hepato-Biliary-Pancreat Surg. 1994;1(2):145–51.

2

Indications for Cholangioscopy, Pre-procedural Patient Care and Preparation

Indications

Cholangioscopy facilitates direct examination of the bile duct and is indicated in:

1. Facilitating lithotripsy of ductal stones
2. The evaluation of indeterminate biliary strictures
3. Retrieval of migrated stents and other foreign bodies form the bile duct
4. Facilitating guidewire and device access across tight biliary strictures

Cholangioscopy is principally used in the management of bile duct stones that are difficult to remove using conventional stone extraction methods, including mechanical lithotripsy [1–6]. Cholangioscopy facilitates the application of electrohydraulic lithotripsy (EHL) or laser lithotripsy to achieve fragmentation of stones, thereby aiding stone extraction and duct clearance [5, 7–11]. The platform used to perform cholangioscopy can additionally be used to access the pancreatic duct (pancreatoscopy) and treat pancreatic duct stones. In addition to treating stone disease, cholangioscopy and pancreatoscopy can be used to evaluate the biliary and pancreatic systems to identify, examine and sample biliary and pancreatic strictures [12–40]. Cholangioscopy and pancreatoscopy can be used to retrieve migrated stents from the bile duct or pancreatic duct when other extraction techniques have failed and can be used to direct and facilitate guidewire access across tight biliary strictures [41–49]. The utility and range of cholangioscopic platforms have rapidly expanded due to improvements in their imaging capabilities and therapeutic ability. These systems have integrated with other tools in the armamentarium of a hepatobiliary endoscopist.

Pre-procedural Patient Care and Preparation

Preparation for endoscopic retrograde cholangiopancreatography (ERCP) generally involves no food intake for 4–8 h, although clear fluids can be consumed up to 2 h prior to the procedure [50, 51].

Consent

Patients should be counselled about the risks and benefits of ERCP in advance. Cholangioscopy confers additional procedure-related risks of infection and bleeding and procedure leaflets with information pertaining, to ERCP in general, with a specific section on cholangioscopy serve as a useful tool to inform patients [19, 52]. Written, informed consent should be taken in advance for all elective procedures and patients should be allowed enough time to consider the information provided to them in order to make an informed decision.

Pre-assessment

When a clinical decision is made to undertake ERCP with cholangioscopy, a thorough pre-assessment is important. The following issues should be evaluated and addressed during pre-assessment:

1. *Risk of bleeding*
   Complete blood examination and coagulation profile should be obtained and assessed for the haemoglobin level, platelet count and International Normalized Ratio (INR). A platelet count of $>50 \times 10^9$/l and INR of <1.5 are important pre-requisites for any therapeutic endoscopy. Anticoagulants and antiplatelets will generally need to be stopped prior to cholangioscopy owing to the risk of bleeding related to a sphincterotomy which is necessary for cholangioscopic access, and due to techniques likely to increase the risk of bleeding, such as sphincteroplasty and lithotripsy which may cause duct-wall injury. The risk of stopping anticoagulant and antiplatelet therapy needs to be balanced against the risk of thromboembolic events and detailed guidance on managing anticoagulant and antiplatelet therapy for diagnostic and therapeutic endoscopy has been published by the British Society of Gastroenterology (BSG) [53]. These have been summarised in Tables 2.1 and 2.2.
2. *Cardiopulmonary status*
   Patients with cardiac and pulmonary disease may need optimisation of cardiopulmonary status before ERCP with cholangioscopy owing to a potentially longer procedure time and greater risk of cardiopulmonary complications. Moreover, general anaesthesia (as opposed to

Table 2.1 Guidelines for management of patients on anticoagulant agents undergoing ERCP

Drugs	Low risk conditions	High risk conditions
	Prosthetic aortic valve, xenograft heart valve, atrial fibrillation (AF) without valvular disease, >3 months after venous thromboembolism (VTE)	Prosthetic metal mitral valve, prosthetic heart valve and AF, AF and mitral stenosis, <3 months after VTE
Warfarin	Stop 5 days before	Stop 5 days before. Start *LMWH 2 days after stopping warfarin. Last dose >24 h before the procedure
Direct oral anticoagulants (Dabigatran, Rivaroxaban, Apixaban, Edoxaban)	Last dose >48 h before ERCP For Dabigatran: if ¶eGFR 30–50 ml/min, last dose >72 h before procedure	

LMWH low molecular weight heparin; *eGFR* estimated glomerular filtration rate

deep sedation or monitored anaesthesia with Propofol) may be necessary for cholangioscopy with lithotripsy.

3. *Allergy status*

   Frequently used medications during ERCP include sedatives/anaesthetic agents, antibiotics and non-steroidal anti-inflammatory drug (NSAID) suppositories. Any drug allergies should be documented and should prompt use of alternatives.

4. *Airway issues*

   Cholangioscopy generally involves deep sedation/anaesthesia and any airway-associated issues need to be identified in advance. A pre-procedural anaesthetic assessment is an important aspect of planning and patient-preparation.

Table 2.2 Guidelines for management of patients on antiplatelet agents undergoing ERCP

Drugs	Low risk conditions	High risk conditions
Aspirin	Ischaemic heart disease without stents, cerebrovascular disease, peripheral vascular disease Continue	Coronary artery stents Continue
Clopidogrel Ticagrelor Prasugrel	Stop 5 days before ERCP	Liaise with cardiologist Consider stopping 5 days before if >12 months after insertion of drug-eluting coronary stents, and >1 month after insertion of bare metal stent

5. *Radiation exposure*

ERCP involves use of X-rays in the form of fluoroscopy and cholangioscopy may lead to a longer period of fluoroscopic screening. Patients should be made aware of this issue and women of reproductive age should be asked for possibility of pregnancy. A pregnancy test may need to be performed pre-procedure.

Procedural Considerations

1. *Endoscopy safety checklist*

A safety checklist should be performed for every patient before the start of the procedure. The World Health Organization (WHO) checklist was initially developed to reduce the adverse events from surgical procedures [54]. A safety checklist comprises two steps: an initial 'time out', when key information regarding the patient and procedure at hand are confirmed before starting endoscopy and a subsequent 'sign out' at the end of procedure confirming specimens, the endoscopy report and follow up plans.

2. *Team Brief*

   A team brief before the start of the list helps to prepare the endoscopy team for the procedure and patient specific and equipment related issues should be discussed with an outline of planned therapy. The following should be discussed:

   (a) *Patient position*

   ERCP is generally performed in the prone position. Airway management is particularly important in the supine position owing to risk of aspiration.

   (b) *Accessories*

   Endoscopic accessories needed for cholangioscopy should be discussed and identified as part of the team briefing. Radio-opaque contrast syringes should be prepared, and strength of the dye should be decided to suit the indication and endoscopist preference. Full strength contrast is used to delineate strictures and pancreatic duct anatomy, while half-strength contrast is more suitable to visualise duct stones [55].

   (c) *Endoscopic non-technical skills*

   Non-technical skills such as communication, decision-making, leadership and situation awareness are increasingly recognised as being central to effective functioning of the endoscopy team [56]. Good communication and coordination between the team members is important to ensure patient safety, prevent errors and lead to better patient outcomes.

3. *Radiation exposure to staff*

   ERCP utilises X-rays in the form of fluoroscopy. Appropriate measures should be taken to reduce the radiation exposure to staff. Limiting the duration of exposure, keeping a reasonable distance from radiation source and lead shielding helps to keep the overall incident radiation 'As Low as Reasonably Achievable'. This is known as the ALARA principle [57].

4. *Medications used in ERCP*
   (a) *Sedation/anaesthesia*

   Owing to longer procedure time for cholangioscopy, deep sedation/anaesthesia is required, and anaesthetic assistance is important. Nursing staff managing the airway need to be vigilant about the potential for respiratory depression/airway compromise if cholangioscopy is being performed with sedation.

   (b) *Anti-spasmodic drugs*

   Duodenal contractions can make cannulation of the ampulla difficult. Hyoscine is usually used as an anti-spasmodic to aid cannulation owing to its anticholinergic effects. Care should be exercised in patients with significant cardiac issues and cardiac arrhythmias [58]. Intravenous Glucagon is an alternative to Hyoscine in non-diabetic patients.

   (c) *Antibiotics*

   Most patients undergoing conventional ERCP do not require antibiotics. However, cholangioscopy is a complex procedure with risk of cholangitis and antibiotic prophylaxis should be considered [59, 60].

   (d) *Rectal Non-Steroidal Anti-Inflammatory Drugs (NSAIDs)*

   Rectal NSAIDs (100 mg of indomethacin or diclofenac via the rectal route before or immediately after ERCP) should be considered to reduce the risk of post ERCP pancreatitis (PEP) [61, 62].

Post-procedural Care

Following ERCP and cholangioscopy, patients should be monitored for at least 3–4 h to ensure safe recovery from sedation/anaesthesia and development of any early signs of post-ERCP complications. Severe abdominal pain, hypotension and tachypnoea should prompt a review. Clear instructions pertaining to resuming a diet, need for antibiotics on discharge and when to resume antiplatelet/anticoagulation drugs should be part of post-procedural care. The results of the procedure should be conveyed to the patients and patients should be provided with aftercare information with points of contact in case of any concern.

ERCP and Pacemakers/Defibrillators

Special consideration has to be given to patients with implanted cardiac devices [pacemaker or implantable cardiac defibrillators (ICD)]. As these devices are designed to detect electrical impulses, use of electrocautery during ERCP carries a risk of electrical interference. This is particularly an issue with ICDs where current from electrocautery can potentially result in discharging of the device. The following precautions hence need to be taken to minimise any stimulation of the cardiac device [63]:

(a) Minimise use of electrocautery and apply the electrocautery plate on the patient as far away from the cardiac device as possible
(b) Ensure cardiac monitoring during the procedure
(c) Cardiac physiology review during pre-assessment if appropriate (particularly for ICDs)
(d) Use of a magnet over the pacemaker/ICD to disable its sensory function and undertake pacing at a fixed rhythm.

Example Patient Information Leaflet

This is a sample patient information leaflet used at the senior authors' institution.

What Is an ERCP?

Endoscopic Retrograde Cholangio Pancreatography (ERCP) is a procedure that allows the endoscopist to examine the tubes (ducts) that drain bile from your liver and gallbladder and digestive juices from the pancreas. To do this a flexible endoscope is passed into the mouth, through the oesophagus (gullet), stomach to the duodenum to find the small opening called Ampulla of Vater where the bile and digestive juices drain into the intestine. A thin tube is then passed through the endoscope and up into the Ampulla so that dye can be injected, and X-Rays are then taken.

In most cases a small incision is made in the ampulla to help relieve an obstruction in the ducts. This is called a sphincterotomy. In other cases, a tube called a stent is placed into an area where the bile duct is blocked to allow the bile to drain.

A biopsy (small sample of tissue) of the ducts is sometimes also required. Any samples taken will be sent to the laboratory for analysis. An ERCP usually takes 30–40 min but times vary considerably.

Why Do I Need to Have an ERCP?

The gallbladder lies under the liver on the right side of the upper abdomen. It stores bile between meals. It contracts (squeezes) when you eat, emptying stored bile back into the bile duct. The pancreas is a large gland that makes enzymes (chemicals) which are vital to digest food. Jaundice (yellowing of the skin and urine) occurs when the tubes draining the bile become blocked. In most cases ERCP is performed to try and relieve obstruction in the ducts either due to gallstones or narrowing of the ducts.

What Are the Risks of ERCP?

As with all medical procedures there are clearly defined risks involved. The doctor who has requested the test will have considered these risks and compared them to the benefit of having the procedures carried out.
The main risks are:

- **Pancreatitis** Inflammation of the pancreas gland. Pancreatitis is painful and would require admission to hospital for treatment. The severity of this condition is variable. The risk of pancreatitis is 5%.
- **Infection** in the bile ducts. An infection in the biliary tree would require admission into hospital for treatment with fluids and antibiotics. The risk of infection is 2%.
- **Bleeding** may occur at the site of a sphincterotomy. It can usually be controlled by treatment through the endoscope. A blood transfusion may be required occasionally. The risk of bleeding is 2%.
- **Perforation** (tear) of the lining of the digestive tract. A perforation would require admission to hospital for treatment with fluids and antibiotics and might require surgery to repair the tear. The risk of perforation is 1%.

What Is Per Oral Cholangioscopy?

Per oral Cholangioscopy (POC) is an important tool for diagnosis and treatment of various biliary disorders. Conventional ERCP provides X-ray images only. This technology enables the endoscopist to directly view the bile duct. POC can be performed by using a dedicated cholangioscope (slim flexible disposable scope) that is inserted through the accessory channel of the flexible endoscope into the bile duct for direct visualization. This system provides the endoscopist with direct vision of the bile ducts for diagnostic and therapeutic applications. The disposable digital cholangioscope is designed to optimize procedural outcomes for patients with indeterminate strictures (unknown cause of narrowing in the bile ducts) or large difficult stones in the bile duct.

What Is Cholangioscopy Used For?

This technology can be used to help improve the diagnosis of indeterminate strictures in the bile ducts, and therapy for complex bile duct stones.

Strictures in the Bile Ducts

When conventional methods of diagnosing the nature of strictures in the bile duct prove inconclusive, POC can be used to directly view the abnormality and also allow the endoscopist to take targeted biopsies via the cholangioscope, helping with diagnostic accuracy.

Stones in the Bile Ducts

Sometimes stones in the bile duct cannot be removed via conventional ERCP due to reasons such as size, quantity, shape or ductal anatomy. POC has a therapeutic application whereby complex bile duct stones can be broken up using electrohydraulic lithotripsy (EHL) or laser therapy under direct vision.

Preparing for Your Procedure

It is important to have clear views during the ERCP, and for this the stomach must be empty. In most cases you must not eat anything for 4–6 h before the procedure. You can drink water only up to 2 h before the procedure. The team at your hospital will provide more detail regarding the preparation for your procedure.

What Will Happen After the Procedure?

You will be taken to the recovery area. Your blood pressure and heart rate will be monitored. You will remain fasting following the procedure. Direct instructions will be given regarding your post procedure care from the medical team looking after you.

Are There Any Increased Risks with Cholangioscopy?

The risks are very similar to that of ERCP. There may be a slight increase in the risk of infection depending on the reason why you are having the cholangioscopy procedure.

Your Doctor may give you an extended course of antibiotic cover as appropriate.

References

1. Chen YK, et al. Single-operator cholangioscopy in patients requiring evaluation of bile duct disease or therapy of biliary stones (with videos). Gastrointest Endosc. 2011;74(4):805–14.
2. Committee AT, et al. Cholangiopancreatoscopy. Gastrointest Endosc. 2008;68(3):411–21.
3. Piraka C, et al. Transpapillary cholangioscopy-directed lithotripsy in patients with difficult bile duct stones. Clin Gastroenterol Hepatol. 2007;5(11):1333–8.
4. Arya N, et al. Electrohydraulic lithotripsy in 111 patients: a safe and effective therapy for difficult bile duct stones. Am J Gastroenterol. 2004;99(12):2330–4.
5. Brown NG, et al. Advanced ERCP techniques for the extraction of complex biliary stones: a single referral center's 12-year experience. Scand J Gastroenterol. 2018;53(5):626–31.
6. Brauer BC, Shah RJ. Cholangioscopy in liver disease. Clin Liver Dis. 2014;18(4):927–44.
7. Committee AT, et al. Biliary and pancreatic lithotripsy devices. VideoGIE. 2018;3(11):329–38.
8. Nourani S, Haber G. Cholangiopancreatoscopy: a comprehensive review. Gastrointest Endosc Clin N Am. 2009;19(4):527–43.
9. Kamiyama R, et al. Electrohydraulic lithotripsy for difficult bile duct stones under endoscopic retrograde cholangiopancreatography and peroral transluminal cholangioscopy guidance. Gut Liver. 2018;12(4):457–62.
10. Jones JD, Pawa R. Single-operator peroral cholangioscopy for extraction of cystic duct stones in postcholecystectomy Mirizzi syndrome. Case Rep Gastrointest Med. 2017;2017:1710501.

11. Anjum MR, et al. Cholangioscopy-guided electrohydraulic lithotripsy of a large bile duct stone through a percutaneous T-tube tract. VideoGIE. 2018;3(12):390–1.
12. Ayoub F, Yang D, Draganov PV. Cholangioscopy in the digital era. Transl Gastroenterol Hepatol. 2018;3:82.
13. Tabibian JH, et al. Advanced endoscopic imaging of indeterminate biliary strictures. World J Gastrointest Endosc. 2015;7(18):1268–78.
14. Gabbert C, et al. Advanced techniques for endoscopic biliary imaging: cholangioscopy, endoscopic ultrasonography, confocal, and beyond. Gastrointest Endosc Clin N Am. 2013;23(3):625–46.
15. Franzini TA, Moura RN, de Moura EG. Advances in therapeutic cholangioscopy. Gastroenterol Res Pract. 2016;2016:5249152.
16. Navaneethan U, Moon JH, Itoi T. Biliary interventions using single operator cholangioscopy. Dig Endosc. 2019.
17. Singh A, Gelrud A, Agarwal B. Biliary strictures: diagnostic considerations and approach. Gastroenterol Rep (Oxf). 2015;3(1):22–31.
18. Khan AH, et al. Cholangiopancreatoscopy and endoscopic ultrasound for indeterminate pancreaticobiliary pathology. Dig Dis Sci. 2013;58(4):1110–5.
19. Darcy M, Picus D. Cholangioscopy. Tech Vasc Interv Radiol. 2008;11(2):133–42.
20. Moura EG, et al. Cholangioscopy in bile duct disease: a case series. Arq Gastroenterol. 2014;51(3):250–4.
21. Ross AS, Kozarek RA. Cholangioscopy: where are we now? Curr Opin Gastroenterol. 2009;25(3):245–51.
22. Ren X, et al. Co-occurrence of IPMN and malignant IPNB complicated by a pancreatobiliary fistula: a case report and review of the literature. World J Clin Cases. 2019;7(1):102–8.
23. Parsi MA, et al. Diagnostic and therapeutic cholangiopancreatoscopy: performance of a new digital cholangioscope. Gastrointest Endosc. 2014;79(6):936–42.

24. Kurihara T, et al. Diagnostic and therapeutic single-operator cholangiopancreatoscopy in biliopancreatic diseases: prospective multicenter study in Japan. World J Gastroenterol. 2016;22(5):1891–901.
25. Kalaitzakis E, et al. Diagnostic and therapeutic utility of single-operator peroral cholangioscopy for indeterminate biliary lesions and bile duct stones. Eur J Gastroenterol Hepatol. 2012;24(6):656–64.
26. Tieu AH, et al. Diagnostic and therapeutic utility of SpyGlass((R)) peroral cholangioscopy in intraductal biliary disease: single-center, retrospective, cohort study. Dig Endosc. 2015;27(4):479–85.
27. Navaneethan U, et al. Digital, single-operator cholangiopancreatoscopy in the diagnosis and management of pancreatobiliary disorders: a multicenter clinical experience (with video). Gastrointest Endosc. 2016;84(4):649–55.
28. Pereira P, et al. How SpyGlass may impact endoscopic retrograde cholangiopancreatography practice and patient management. GE Port J Gastroenterol. 2018;25(3):132–7.
29. Siddiqui AA, et al. Identification of cholangiocarcinoma by using the Spyglass Spyscope system for peroral cholangioscopy and biopsy collection. Clin Gastroenterol Hepatol. 2012;10(5):466–71; quiz e48.
30. Varadarajulu S, et al. Improving the diagnostic yield of single-operator cholangioscopy-guided biopsy of indeterminate biliary strictures: ROSE to the rescue? (with video). Gastrointest Endosc. 2016;84(4):681–7.
31. Walter D, Hartmann S, Albert JG. Indeterminate biliary stricture with suspicion for malignancy unmasked as eosinophilic cholangitis by cholangioscopy. Gastrointest Endosc. 2017;85(1):265–6.
32. Tringali A, et al. Intraductal biliopancreatic imaging: European Society of Gastrointestinal Endoscopy (ESGE) technology review. Endoscopy. 2015;47(8):739–53.
33. Walter D, et al. Intraductal biopsies in indeterminate biliary stricture: evaluation of histopathological criteria in fluoroscopy- vs. cholangioscopy guided technique. Dig Liver Dis. 2016;48(7):765–70.

34. Sun X, et al. Is single-operator peroral cholangioscopy a useful tool for the diagnosis of indeterminate biliary lesion? A systematic review and meta-analysis. Gastrointest Endosc. 2015;82(1):79–87.
35. Figueroa Marrero A, et al. Long-standing indeterminate biliary stricture with iterative negative tissue sampling revealed as cholangiocarcinoma under SpyGlassTM cholangioscopy. Rev Esp Enferm Dig. 2017;109(3):220–1.
36. Ramchandani M, et al. Role of single-operator peroral cholangioscopy in the diagnosis of indeterminate biliary lesions: a single-center, prospective study. Gastrointest Endosc. 2011;74(3):511–9.
37. Woo YS, et al. Role of SpyGlass peroral cholangioscopy in the evaluation of indeterminate biliary lesions. Dig Dis Sci. 2014;59(10):2565–70.
38. Hartman DJ, et al. Tissue yield and diagnostic efficacy of fluoroscopic and cholangioscopic techniques to assess indeterminate biliary strictures. Clin Gastroenterol Hepatol. 2012;10(9):1042–6.
39. Williamson JB, Draganov PV. The usefulness of SpyGlass choledochoscopy in the diagnosis and treatment of biliary disorders. Curr Gastroenterol Rep. 2012;14(6):534–41.
40. Laleman W, et al. Usefulness of the single-operator cholangioscopy system SpyGlass in biliary disease: a single-center prospective cohort study and aggregated review. Surg Endosc. 2017;31(5):2223–32.
41. Bokemeyer A, et al. Digital single-operator cholangioscopy: a useful tool for selective guidewire placements across complex biliary strictures. Surg Endosc. 2018.
42. Akerman S, Rahman M, Bernstein DE. Direct cholangioscopy: the North Shore experience. Eur J Gastroenterol Hepatol. 2012;24(12):1406–9.
43. Ogura T, et al. Migrated endoclip removal after cholecystectomy under digital single-operator cholangioscopy guidance. Endoscopy. 2018;50(3):E74–5.

44. Sanaka MR, Wadhwa V, Patel M. Retrieval of proximally migrated biliary stent with direct peroral cholangioscopy with an ultraslim endoscope. Gastrointest Endosc. 2015;81(6):1483–4.
45. Rahimi A, Ejtehadi F. SpyGlass pancreatoscopy and successful retrieval of a proximally migrated pancreatic stent; unusual case and technical tips. Middle East J Dig Dis. 2016;8(3):232–4.
46. Ogura T, et al. Successful digital cholangioscopy removal of a stent-retriever tip migrated into the periphery of the bile duct. Endoscopy. 2018;50(5):E113–4.
47. Banerjee D, et al. Successful removal of proximally migrated biliary stent in a liver transplant patient by single-operator digital cholangioscopy. ACG Case Rep J. 2018;5:e50.
48. Kantsevoy SV, Frolova EA, Thuluvath PJ. Successful removal of the proximally migrated pancreatic winged stent by using the SpyGlass visualization system. Gastrointest Endosc. 2010;72(2):454–5.
49. Menon S, Holt A. Digital cholangioscopic evaluation of a post-liver transplantation stricture. VideoGIE. 2018;28(3):81–2.
50. Faigel DO, et al. Preparation of patients for GI endoscopy. Gastrointest Endosc. 2003;57(4):446–50.
51. American Society of Anesthesiologists C. Practice guidelines for preoperative fasting and the use of pharmacologic agents to reduce the risk of pulmonary aspiration: application to healthy patients undergoing elective procedures: an updated report by the American Society of Anesthesiologists Committee on Standards and Practice Parameters. Anesthesiology 2011;114(3):495–511.
52. Tanaka R, et al. New digital cholangiopancreatoscopy for diagnosis and therapy of pancreaticobiliary diseases (with videos). J Hepatobiliary Pancreat Sci. 2016;23(4):220–6.
53. Veitch AM, et al. Endoscopy in patients on antiplatelet or anticoagulant therapy, including direct oral anticoagulants: British Society of Gastroenterology (BSG) and European Society of Gastrointestinal Endoscopy (ESGE) guidelines. Gut. 2016;65(3):374–89.

54. Haynes AB, et al. A surgical safety checklist to reduce morbidity and mortality in a global population. N Engl J Med. 2009;360(5):491–9.
55. Mishkin D, et al. ASGE Technology Status Evaluation Report: radiographic contrast media used in ERCP. Gastrointest Endosc. 2005;62(4):480–4.
56. Matharoo M, et al. Endoscopic non-technical skills team training: the next step in quality assurance of endoscopy training. World J Gastroenterol. 2014;20(46):17507–15.
57. Uffmann M, Schaefer-Prokop C. Digital radiography: the balance between image quality and required radiation dose. Eur J Radiol. 2009;72(2):202–8.
58. Ozaslan E, Karakelle N, Ozaslan NG. Hyoscine-N-butylbromide induced ventricular tachycardia during ERCP. J Anaesthesiol Clin Pharmacol. 2014;30(1):118–9.
59. Adler DG. Cholangioscopy, cholangitis, and antibiotics: a tale of bugs and drugs. Gastrointest Endosc. 2016;83(1):158–9.
60. Sethi A, et al. ERCP with cholangiopancreatoscopy may be associated with higher rates of complications than ERCP alone: a single-center experience. Gastrointest Endosc. 2011;73(2):251–6.
61. Elmunzer BJ, et al. A randomized trial of rectal indomethacin to prevent post-ERCP pancreatitis. N Engl J Med. 2012;366(15):1414–22.
62. Dumonceau JM, et al. Prophylaxis of post-ERCP pancreatitis: European Society of Gastrointestinal Endoscopy (ESGE) Guideline—updated June 2014. Endoscopy. 2014;46(9):799–815.
63. Petersen BT, et al. Endoscopy in patients with implanted electronic devices. Gastrointest Endosc. 2007;65(4):561–8.

3

Single Operator Cholangioscopy

Boston Scientific (Boston Scientific Corporation, USA) developed a fibreoptic cholangioscopy platform in 2007 called Spyglass™ that revolutionized single operator cholangioscopy. This system included a cholangioscopy catheter that could be introduced through the working channel of a duodenoscope (over a guidewire) and strapped onto the side of the duodenoscope using a silastic strap, a pump to provide irrigation (sterile saline/water) and disposable devices that could be introduced through an instrumentation channel on the cholangioscope. The cholangioscope itself was a 10 Fr disposable 4-lumen catheter (Cholangioscope) with a 0.9 mm channel for the fibreoptic probe, a 1.2 mm channel to pass instruments/accessories and two 0.6 mm irrigation channels. A 3 Fr disposable biopsy forceps (SpyBite™) was available with the system and could be passed down the cholangioscope.

Electronic supplementary material The online version of this chapter (https://doi.org/10.1007/978-3-030-27261-6_3) contains supplementary material, which is available to authorized users.

Fibres to facilitate electrohydraulic lithotripsy (EHL) or laser lithotripsy could be additionally passed down the cholangioscope. The cholangioscope had 4-way tip deflection that facilitated manoeuvrability within the pancreaticobiliary system. The fibreoptic system was upgraded to a digital SpyGlass™ DS in 2007 and more recently, a further upgrade to a 3rd generation system called the SpyGlass™ DS II was launched [1]. The SpyGlass™ DS and DS II systems are single-use 10 Fr cholangioscopes and represent a significant improvement in image resolution in comparison to the legacy fibreoptic system. These digital cholangioscopes have retained the basic features of the legacy cholangioscope, with two irrigation channels and an instrumentation channel, and have a simple 'plug-and-play' setup onto a processor. Boston Scientific partnered with Northgate Technologies Inc (USA) in 2017 to distribute Northgate's EHL system called Autolith™. The Autolith™ system delivers energy to facilitate EHL through a 1.9 Fr disposable probe. In 2018, Boston Scientific released a retrieval basket and snare with the SpyGlass™ DS II system.

The set up and technique described in this chapter relates to the digital SpyGlass platforms.

Cholangioscopy Technique

Please see online Video A that demonstrates the set-up, monitoring and use of the SpyGlass single operator cholangioscopy system.

The digital cholangioscope is generally inserted over a 450 cm guidewire that is initially placed in the pancreaticobiliary system at ERCP. Standard ERCP techniques are used for cannulation and duct access following which 'long-wire' (450 cm guidewire) access is achieved for biliary endotherapy. A biliary sphincterotomy is generally necessary to facilitate the advancement of the cholangioscope into the bile duct. A sphincterotomy additionally mitigates against increases in hydrostatic pressures in the biliary system by allowing flow around the cholangioscope. The cholangioscope is supplied in a sterile box and is assembled by plugging its cable onto the SpyGlass DS processor. The cholangioscope has an irrigation cable which is connected onto an irrigation pump generally delivering sterile saline and a separate suction cable with a three-way connector, which can be connected to a suction system. The processor and monitor are delivered on a dedicated stack that houses the Autolith™ generator and the cabling for the SpyGlass system.

The cholangioscope is advanced over the guidewire into the biliary system and is strapped onto the side of the duodenoscope. The cholangioscope sits just underneath and slightly to the right of the duodenoscope instrument channel. The duodenoscope position is stabilised once the cholangioscope is advanced out of the duodenoscope. Plugging the cholangioscope immediately generates a digital image on the SpyGlass monitor with the light on the cholangioscope activated. The light is generally turned off in order to reduce glare and facilitate visibility whilst advancing the scope into the bile duct. Advancement of the cholangioscope into the distal bile duct is generally easy over a guidewire, although freehand cannulation across a wide, sphincterotomised papillary orifice is also feasible. The cholangioscope has a single lock for its wheels, which can be applied to stabilise the tip and prevent excessive deflection. Advancement into the proximal bile duct is facilitated by a combination of insertion of the cholangioscope, adjustment of wheels and irrigation using the foot pump to aid visualisation. Once the cholangioscope is stabilised adjacent to a target (stone, stricture, etc.), the guidewire is removed to facilitate the deployment of accessories for therapy. Deep sedation or anaesthesia is generally required to facilitate cholangioscopy and lithotripsy.

Lithotripsy

Lithotripsy or fragmentation of stones is carried out using electrohydraulic lithotripsy or laser lithotripsy.

Electrohydraulic Lithotripsy (EHL)

Please see online Video cases 1–7 and 11 that demonstrate the use of EHL to fragment stones in the bile duct.

The principle of EHL is the creation of shock waves in a fluid column that delivers energy needed for stone fragmentation [2, 3]. Shock waves are created following the delivery of a rapid electric discharge centred at the tip of a probe. This generates a spark 'plasma' and the resultant development and implosion of a 'cavitation bubble' creates shock waves that deliver energy. EHL is delivered using a 1.9 mm probe inserted through the cholangioscope [4]. Once a stable position has been achieved in the bile duct, the guidewire is withdrawn from the cholangioscope and the EHL probe is inserted. Delivering the EHL probe out of the cholangioscope into the bile duct may be occasionally challenging due to friction within the accessory channel of the cholangioscope and manipulation of the scope (either inserting further into the duct or withdrawing it slightly) and/or releasing the elevator of the duodenoscope facilitates insertion of the EHL probe around the duodenal angle of the duodenoscope and into the bile duct.

The tip of the EHL probe (seen at the 6 O'clock position on the cholangioscopic view) is then positioned adjacent to the stone in order to provide a fluid cushion between the tip of the probe and the stone. This fluid cushion serves to create shock waves. Care must be taken to not be too close to the stone to prevent damage to the cholangioscope. The EHL probe is connected to the Autolith™ generator to deliver energy. The Autolith™ Touch [4] system has three energy settings (low/medium/high: equating to 70–100 W) and different pulse settings (5, 15, 30 pulses). The pulse settings represent the number of pulses of energy delivered by a single activation of a foot pedal that controls the delivery of energy. Generally, energy and pulse settings are set low and are increased progressively depending on the lithotripsy effect. Saline is irrigated into the duct to provide a fluid column and lithotripsy is performed by pressing on the foot pedal of the Autolith™ system. Delivery of energy is seen as rapid pulses observed on the cholangioscopic view and stone fragmentation is observed in real time. Lithotripsy is continued by progressive application of energy across fracture points within the stone surface or by applying energy directly onto stone fragments to break these down to smaller pieces. This is enabled by manoeuvring the cholangioscope within the duct. EHL can cause trauma to the bile duct wall resulting in a risk of bleeding or perforation, so care must be taken to avoid being too close to the duct wall. Stone fragmentation can result in poor visibility and may need removal of the cholangioscope over the wire and the use of stone removal techniques using balloons or baskets to deliver fragments prior to successive sequences of lithotripsy. The process is iterative until stone fragmentation and duct clearance is achieved (Figs. 3.1, 3.2 and 3.3).

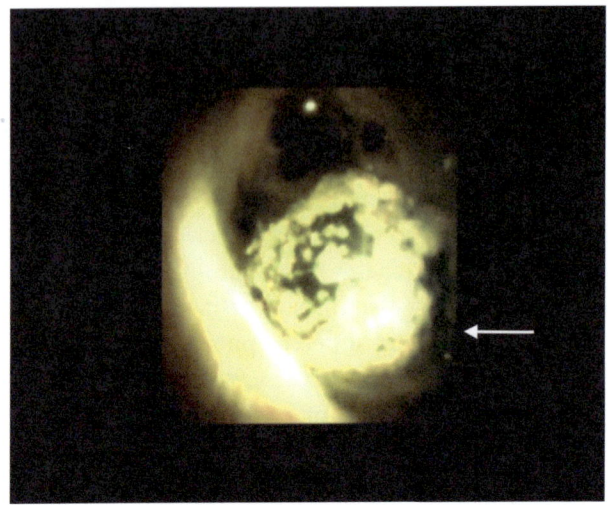

Fig. 3.1 Small intrahepatic duct stone (arrow)

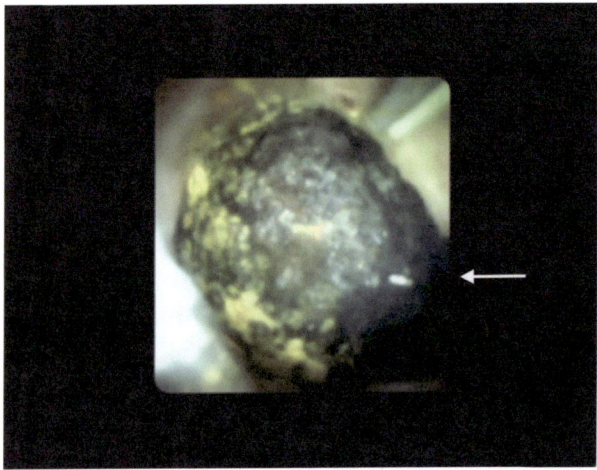

Fig. 3.2 Ductal stone (arrow) accessed via a T-tube in a patient post antrectomy for gastric cancer and who underwent cholecystectomy

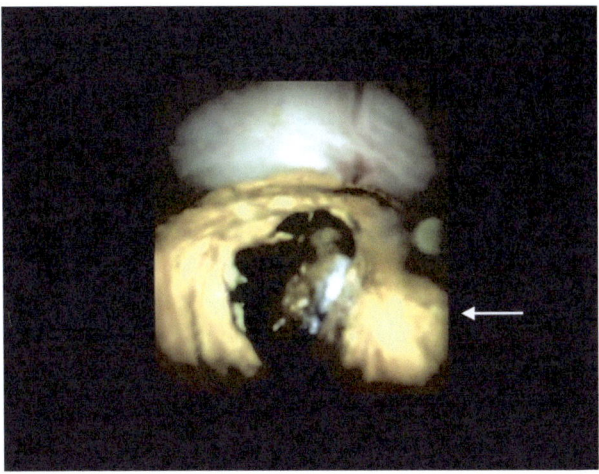

Fig. 3.3 Stone fragment (arrow) post EHL

Laser Lithotripsy

Laser lithotripsy is performed using the Holmium laser, commonly used to treat renal stones. The energy applied is 0.2–0.6 J, with frequencies of 15–50 Hz [5], and can produce a deeper delivery of energy compared to EHL. Contact and non-contact techniques are applied depending on the size of the stone/fragment to either fragment stones into pieces by drilling into the stone using contact techniques or pulverize them with non-contact techniques.

Both EHL and Laser lithotripsy have efficacy rates of clearing difficult bile duct stones of 69–81% in a single session and 97–100% in multiple sessions [6–9].

Biopsies

Please see online Video cases 8–10 that demonstrate the utility of the SpyGlass system in the endoscopic assessment of biliary strictures with a view to tissue acquisition.

The SpyGlass system facilitates tissue acquisition by a 1.2 mm biopsy forceps that is inserted through the therapeutic/wire channel of the Cholangioscope. The distal end of the forceps is stiff and there is generally some resistance as the forceps is advanced across the duodenal angle into the bile duct. Techniques similar to releasing the EHL probe are used to facilitate advancement of the forces out of the scope channel. Forceps can be used to grasp and deliver foreign bodies such as migrated stents although newer snares and baskets have been developed that are compatible with the SpyGlass system and can be used instead of forceps.

Multiple series have demonstrated sensitivities of 89–100% and specificities of 79–96% in evaluating biliary strictures [10–15] (Figs. 3.4, 3.5, 3.6, 3.7, 3.8 and 3.9).

Suction

Adequate mucosal views during cholangioscopy are enabled by irrigation of saline through the cholangioscope. However, irrigation increases the hydrostatic pressure within the ductal system which can cause barotrauma. The SpyGlass DS II system has a suction channel that can mitigate against this issue and suction can be maintained continuously or intermittently by using a three-way connector on the suction apparatus. Moreover, duodenal suction with the duodenoscope generates additional suction which is helpful.

3 Single Operator Cholangioscopy

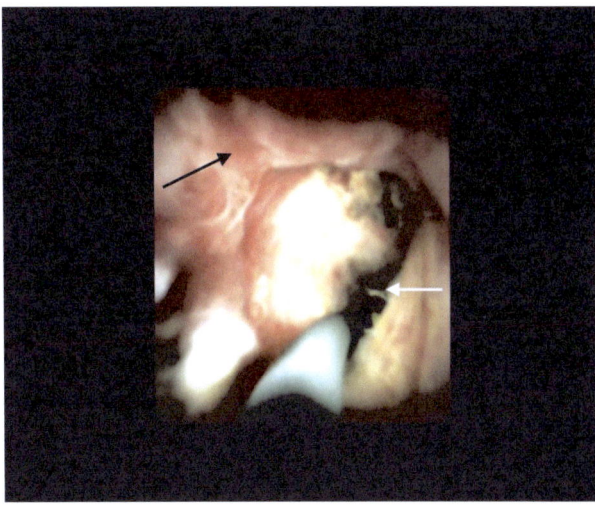

Fig. 3.4 Stricturing tumour of the bile duct (cholangiocarcinoma). A mass lesion is evident (black arrow) with a concurrent bile duct stricture (white arrow) through which a guidewire is seen passing

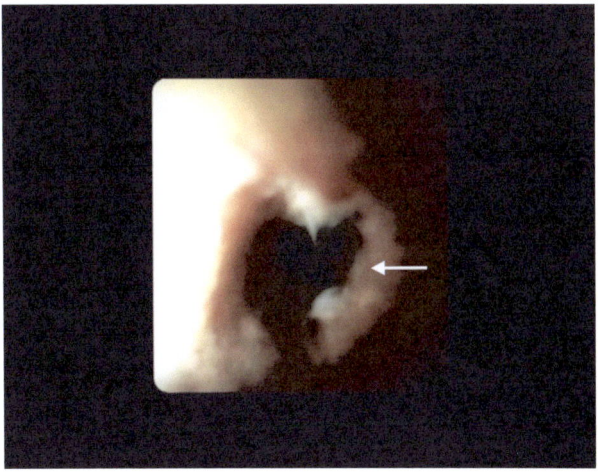

Fig. 3.5 Cholangiocarcinoma associated biliary stricture (arrow)

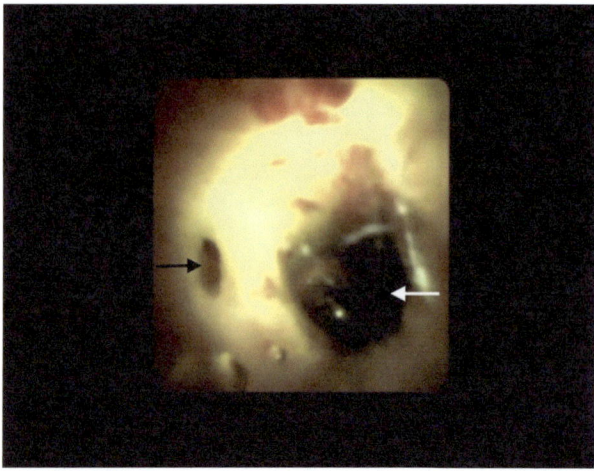

Fig. 3.6 Small diverticulum on the duct wall (black arrow) in a patient with primary sclerosing cholangitis (PSC). A dominant stricture (white arrow) is additionally noted. Biopsies from this stricture confirmed that this was an inflammatory stricture

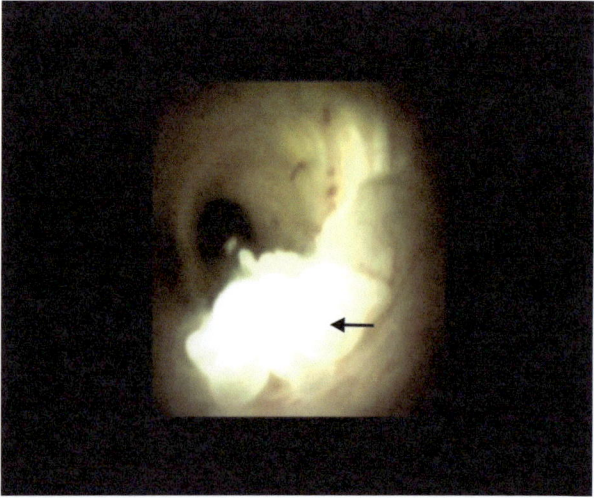

Fig. 3.7 Small biliary wall lesion (arrow). Biopsies revealed inflammatory duct-wall hyperplasia

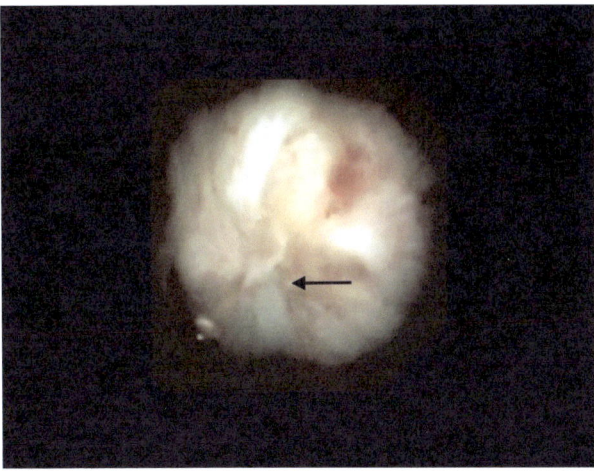

Fig. 3.8 Post liver transplant duct-duct anastomotic stricture with mucin seen extruding from the anastomosis

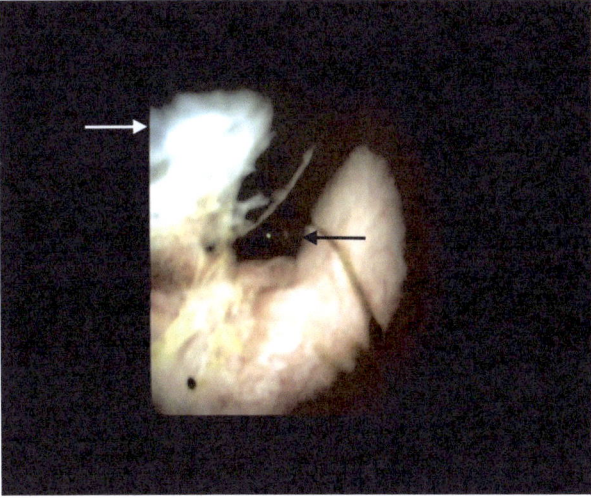

Fig. 3.9 Hydatid cyst seen in the mid-duct (white arrow) in a patient with advanced hydatid disease and cholestasis secondary to cysts causing mechanical obstruction of the biliary lumen. The black arrow indicates the lumen of the bile duct

Complications

The complication rate with cholangioscopy can range from 0 to 25% [7], with the commonest complication being cholangitis (odds ratio (OR) 4.98 [16]), related to ductal irrigation and therefore, post procedure antibiotic cover is important [17–19]. Rates of perforation (OR 3.16) and pancreatitis (OR 1.75) are also higher than in conventional ERCP. Less common complications include haemobilia and bile leaks related to EHL/laser lithotripsy. Cardiorespiratory issues related to deep sedation/anaesthesia are also important, particularly in the setting of prolonged procedures.

Pancreatoscopy

Please see online Video case 12 that demonstrates the use of the SpyGlass system to perform pancreatoscopy and EHL of large stones in the main pancreatic duct in a patient with chronic pancreatitis.

In a similar fashion to cholangioscopy, the SpyGlass system can be inserted into the pancreatic duct to facilitate lithotripsy of stones or less commonly, tissue acquisition. The commonest indication is in the setting of ductal stones in chronic pancreatitis causing symptoms of obstructive pancreatopathy [20]. It does not replace extracorporeal shock wave lithotripsy (ESWL) to fragment pancreatic ductal stones, which is a mature technique with significant efficacy and experience worldwide. Pancreatoscopy may however, be used when access to ESWL is not feasible or if ESWL is not available [21–30]. Techniques for lithotripsy are similar to those applied for bile duct stones. Issues related to this technique relate to access to stones which may be challenging due to the presence of ductal strictures and risks of inducing pancreatitis due to increasing pressures within the pancreatic ductal system during irrigation. Technical success rates of 79–91% and stone clearance rates of 70–88% have been reported with pancreatoscopy-assisted EHL [26, 31], with a complication rate of 10% in one study [25].

References

1. Boston Scientific. SpyGlass™ DS II Direct Visualization System. 2018. https://bsci-prod2-origin.adobecqms.net/content/dam/bostonscientific/endo/portfolio-group/SpyGlass%20DS/SpyGlass-DS-System-ebrochure.pdf.
2. Vorreuther R, Engelmann Y. Evaluation of the shock-wave pattern for endoscopic electrohydraulic lithotripsy. Surg Endosc. 1995;9(1).
3. Manes G, et al. Endoscopic management of common bile duct stones: European Society of Gastrointestinal Endoscopy (ESGE) guideline. Endoscopy. 2019;51(5):472–91.
4. Boston Scientific. Autolith touch biliary EHL system. Boston Scientific; 2018.
5. Aldoukhi AH, et al. Ambulatory tubeless mini-percutaneous nephrolithotomy using Moses technology and dusting technique. Urology. 2018.
6. Chen YK, et al. Single-operator cholangioscopy in patients requiring evaluation of bile duct disease or therapy of biliary stones (with videos). Gastrointest Endosc. 2011;74(4):805–14.
7. Korrapati P, et al. The efficacy of peroral cholangioscopy for difficult bile duct stones and indeterminate strictures: a systematic review and meta-analysis. Endosc Int Open. 2016;4(3):E263–75.

8. Maydeo A, et al. Single-operator cholangioscopy-guided laser lithotripsy in patients with difficult biliary and pancreatic ductal stones (with videos). Gastrointest Endosc. 2011;74(6):1308–14.
9. Farrell JJ, et al. Single-operator duodenoscope-assisted cholangioscopy is an effective alternative in the management of choledocholithiasis not removed by conventional methods, including mechanical lithotripsy. Endoscopy. 2005;37(6):542–7.
10. Siddiqui AA, et al. Identification of cholangiocarcinoma by using the Spyglass Spyscope system for peroral cholangioscopy and biopsy collection. Clin Gastroenterol Hepatol. 2012;10(5):466–71; quiz e48.
11. Sakai Y, et al. Clinical utility of peroral cholangioscopy for mucin-producing bile duct tumor. Hepatogastroenterology. 2008;55(86–87):1509–12.
12. Fukuda Y, et al. Diagnostic utility of peroral cholangioscopy for various bile-duct lesions. Gastrointest Endosc. 2005;62(3):374–82.
13. Sethi A, Shah R. Cholangioscopy and pancreatoscopy. Tech Gastrointest Endosc. 2017;19(3):182–7.
14. Ramchandani M, et al. Per oral cholangiopancreatoscopy in pancreatico biliary diseases–expert consensus statements. World J Gastroenterol. 2015;21(15):4722–34.
15. Rerknimitr R, et al. Asia-Pacific consensus recommendations for endoscopic and interventional management of hilar cholangiocarcinoma. J Gastroenterol Hepatol. 2013;28(4):593–607.
16. Sethi A, et al. ERCP with cholangiopancreatoscopy may be associated with higher rates of complications than ERCP alone: a single-center experience. Gastrointest Endosc. 2011;73(2):251–6.
17. Kalaitzakis E, et al. Diagnostic and therapeutic utility of single-operator peroral cholangioscopy for indeterminate biliary lesions and bile duct stones. Eur J Gastroenterol Hepatol. 2012;24(6):656–64.

18. Brewer Gutierrez OI, et al. Efficacy and safety of digital single-operator cholangioscopy for difficult biliary stones. Clin Gastroenterol Hepatol. 2018;16(6):918–26 e1.
19. Kalaitzakis E, et al. Diagnostic utility of single-user peroral cholangioscopy in sclerosing cholangitis. Scand J Gastroenterol. 2014;49(10):1237–44.
20. Dumonceau JM, et al. Endoscopic treatment of chronic pancreatitis: European Society of Gastrointestinal Endoscopy (ESGE) Clinical Guideline. Endoscopy. 2012;44(8):784–800.
21. Committee AT, et al. Biliary and pancreatic lithotripsy devices. VideoGIE. 2018;3(11):329–38.
22. Alexandrino G, et al. Pancreatoscopy-guided laser lithotripsy in a patient with difficult ductal stone. Endoscopy. 2018;50(6):E130–1.
23. Alexandrino G, et al. Pancreatoscopy-guided electrohydraulic lithotripsy in a patient with calcific chronic pancreatitis. VideoGIE. 2018;3(6):185–6.
24. Ang TL. Chronic pancreatitis with pancreatic duct stricture and calculi treated by fully covered self-expandable metal stent placement and intraductal pancreatoscopy-guided laser lithotripsy. Endoscopy. 2017;49(6):E145–6.
25. Attwell AR, et al. Endoscopic retrograde cholangiopancreatography with per oral pancreatoscopy for calcific chronic pancreatitis using endoscope and catheter-based pancreatoscopes: a 10-year single-center experience. Pancreas. 2014;43(2):268–74.
26. Attwell AR, et al. ERCP with per-oral pancreatoscopy-guided laser lithotripsy for calcific chronic pancreatitis: a multicenter U.S. experience. Gastrointest Endosc. 2015;82(2):311–8.
27. Bekkali NL, et al. Pancreatoscopy-directed electrohydraulic lithotripsy for pancreatic ductal stones in painful chronic pancreatitis using SpyGlass. Pancreas. 2017;46(4):528–30.
28. Chen YI, et al. Single-operator pancreatoscopy with electrohydraulic lithotripsy of large pancreatic duct stones in post-Whipple anatomy. Endoscopy. 2016;48(Suppl 1):E280.

29. Judah JR, Draganov PV. Intraductal biliary and pancreatic endoscopy: an expanding scope of possibility. World J Gastroenterol. 2008;14(20):3129–36.
30. Kuftinec G, Zavadski Y, Tejaswi S. Digital pancreatoscopy with electrohydraulic lithotripsy to treat a pancreatic duct stone. VideoGIE. 2017;2(8):205–7.
31. Ogura T, et al. Prospective evaluation of digital single-operator cholangioscope for diagnostic and therapeutic procedures (with videos). Dig Endosc. 2017;29(7):782–9.

4

Direct Cholangioscopy

Direct cholangioscopy involves the insertion of a standard upper endoscope into the bile duct. Despite being reported in 1977 by Urakami [1], the technique did not become popular owing to the technical difficulties associated with direct biliary intubation with a forward-viewing endoscope. There has been recent interest in this technique owing to the popularity of single operator cholangioscopy. Direct cholangioscopy using conventional upper endoscopes offer significantly improved image quality compared to the SOC platform with possibilities of using image enhancement modalities such as the Olympus® narrow band imaging (NBI) or post processing systems such as the Fujinon® Flexible spectral imaging colour enhancement (FICE) and the Pentax® i-scan. Bigger suction and accessory channels with upper endoscopes are an additional and significant advantage over single operator cholangioscopy.

Equipment and Technique

The Olympus® (GIF-XP160, GIF-XP160N and GIF-XP260N) NBI-incorporated slim upper endoscopes with outer diameters of 5.5–5.9 mm and a working channel of 2 mm are used for direct cholangioscopy. Other platforms include the Fujinon® EG-530NW/530N2 FICE enhanced slim scope (also used as a trans-nasal endoscope) with a tip diameter of 5.9 mm and a working channel of 2 mm and the Pentax® EG-1690 K i-scan enhanced ultra-slim gastroscope with a tip diameter of 5.3 mm and a working channel of 2 mm.

Freehand cannulation of the bile duct with a slim gastroscope is technically challenging and is associated with a high failure rate [2]. Other techniques include overtube-assisted direct cholangioscopy and the anchoring-balloon method. Overtube assisted direct cholangioscopy [3, 4] involves the insertion of an overtube into the gastric-antrum/duodenum to prevent looping of the upper endoscope in the stomach. The endoscope is then manoeuvred into the bile duct by twisting and rotational movements. A generous sphincterotomy and/or sphincteroplasty is important in facilitating endoscope access into the bile duct. Advancement of the endoscope into the proximal bile duct is performed by further rotational and pull-back movements. Access into the bile duct is not reliable and maintaining stability and advancing the endoscope into the proximal bile duct can be challenging. Another method of accessing the bile duct using a slim gastroscope involves inserting a duodenoscope first and performing a conventional ERCP in order to insert an 0.025–0.035-in. guidewire into the bile duct. The guidewire is positioned across the hilum and sphincterotomy, followed by balloon sphincteroplasty to 12–15 mm is performed to enable access. The duodenoscope is withdrawn over the wire and the slim gastroscope is advanced over the guidewire to the papilla. An extraction balloon is inserted through the gastroscope into the bile duct over the guidewire and the balloon is inflated proximal to the hilum. Using traction provided by the balloon on the hilum, the slim gastroscope is inserted into the bile duct. This method provides slightly better gastroscope stability compared to the overtube-assisted method. Endoscope insertion and movement involves rotational/torque and push-pull movements.

Applications include high definition biliary imaging, tissue acquisition, intraductal lithotripsy and intraductal polypectomy [5].

Technical success has been reported to be the highest (96%) with the anchoring balloon method, with technical success rates of 93% with the balloon overtube method and 72% with a combination of freehand cannulation and guidewire/anchoring balloon methods [3, 4, 6–11]. Complications include cholangitis (up to 10%) related to duct instrumentation and irrigation [12, 13], haemobilia and bile leaks associated with intraductal lithotripsy [14, 15]. The use of anchoring balloons has been demonstrated to be a risk factor for bile duct perforation in animal models [16]. There has been concern about the risk of air embolism following a case report of a patient developing left hemiparesis following direct cholangioscopy using the anchoring balloon technique [17]. Recent guidance [18] suggests using carbon dioxide (CO_2) instead of air. However, two fatal cases of CO_2 embolism during direct cholangioscopy [19] have highlighted safety issues with direct cholangioscopy using gas (air or CO_2) insufflation.

Developments/Future Applications

Ongoing developments to the single operator cholangioscopy platform include better image definition, bigger accessory channels to facilitate greater tissue acquisition and therapy and the potential to incorporate advanced mucosal imaging capabilities. Biliary and pancreatic endotherapy, with the possibility of resecting small lesions, delivering haemostatic therapy, mapping of lesions to assist with surgery, surveillance of strictures/biliary or pancreatic lesions and facilitating targeted oncological therapy are the possible future applications of single operator cholangioscopy. Its ease of use has clearly revolutionized the field of hepatobiliary endoscopy and ongoing developments represent a paradigm shift in the management of hepatobiliary and pancreatic disease.

References

1. Urakami Y, Seifert E, Butke H. Peroral direct cholangioscopy (PDCS) using routine straight-view endoscope: first report. Endoscopy. 1977;9(1):27–30.
2. Kozarek RA. Direct cholangioscopy and pancreatoscopy at time of endoscopic retrograde cholangiopancreatography. Am J Gastroenterol. 1988;83(1):55–7.
3. Tsou YK, et al. Direct peroral cholangioscopy using an ultraslim endoscope and overtube balloon-assisted technique: a case series. Endoscopy. 2010;42(8):681–4.
4. Choi HJ, et al. Overtube-balloon-assisted direct peroral cholangioscopy by using an ultra-slim upper endoscope (with videos). Gastrointest Endosc. 2009;69(4):935–40.
5. Beyna T, et al. Endobiliary polypectomy of biliary tumor using a prototype dedicated cholangioscope with double-bending technology. VideoGIE. 2018;3(12).

6. Itoi T. Cholangioscopy. In: Jonnalagadda S, editor. Gastrointestinal endoscopy. New York: Springer Science+Business Media; 2015. p. 23–35.
7. Larghi A, Waxman I. Endoscopic direct cholangioscopy by using an ultra-slim upper endoscope: a feasibility study. Gastrointest Endosc. 2006;63(6):853–7.
8. Yasuda I, Itoi T. Recent advances in endoscopic management of difficult bile duct stones. Dig Endosc 2013;25(4):376–85.
9. Moon JH, et al. Direct peroral cholangioscopy using an ultra-slim upper endoscope for the treatment of retained bile duct stones. Am J Gastroenterol. 2009;104(11):2729–33.
10. Pohl J, Ell C. Direct transnasal cholangioscopy with ultraslim endoscopes: a one-step intraductal balloon-guided approach. Gastrointest Endosc. 2011;74(2):309–16.
11. Lee YN, et al. Direct peroral cholangioscopy using an ultraslim upper endoscope for management of residual stones after mechanical lithotripsy for retained common bile duct stones. Endoscopy. 2012;44(9):819–24.
12. Sethi A, Shah R. Cholangioscopy and pancreatoscopy. Tech Gastrointest Endosc. 2017;19(3):182–7.
13. Meves V, Ell C, Pohl J. Efficacy and safety of direct transnasal cholangioscopy with standard ultraslim endoscopes: results of a large cohort study. Gastrointest Endosc. 2014;79(1):88–94.
14. Arya N, et al. Electrohydraulic lithotripsy in 111 patients: a safe and effective therapy for difficult bile duct stones. Am J Gastroenterol. 2004;99(12):2330–4.
15. Sethi A, et al. ERCP with cholangiopancreatoscopy may be associated with higher rates of complications than ERCP alone: a single-center experience. Gastrointest Endosc. 2011;73(2):251–6.
16. Waxman I, et al. Feasibility of a novel system for intraductal balloon-anchored direct peroral cholangioscopy and endotherapy with an ultraslim endoscope (with videos). Gastrointest Endosc. 2010;72(5):1052–6.

17. Efthymiou M, et al. Air embolism complicated by left hemiparesis after direct cholangioscopy with an intraductal balloon anchoring system. Gastrointest Endosc. 2012;75(1):221–3.
18. Tringali A, et al. Intraductal biliopancreatic imaging: European Society of Gastrointestinal Endoscopy (ESGE) technology review. Endoscopy. 2015;47(8):739–53.
19. Hann A, et al. Fatal outcome due to CO_2 emboli during direct cholangioscopy. Gut. 2018;67(8):1378–9.

Video A: Spyglass Cholangioscopy Introduction and Set Up

Procedure Videos

Stones

1. **Video case 1**
   Title: Stone case: EHL
   Summary of the video
   This video demonstrates the management of a large common bile duct stone. The cholangiogram at the start of the video demonstrates a large stone in the distal bile duct with relatively little space around the stone. The EHL probe is noted at the 6 O'clock position in the cholangioscopy image and EHL is performed in rapid pulses. Due to the density of the stone, easy fragmentation is not possible, so the initial cavity on the

surface of the stone induced by EHL is accessed and progressive cavitation is performed using EHL bursts at this point. The fracture line created is then followed by adjusting the line of the EHL probe, and sequential fragmentation of the stone is performed. Smaller fragments created are broken down in the same fashion. Adequate biliary access through a sphincterotomy is essential and we generally undertake a sphincteroplasty if the patient has had a previous sphincterotomy. In this instance, the sphincterotomy was dilated to 12 mm using a controlled radial expansion (CRE) balloon and the video demonstrates the use of a 12 mm extraction balloon to deliver stone fragments out of the sphincterotomy. An occlusion cholangiogram confirms duct clearance.

2. **Video case 2**
   Title: Stone case 2: EHL
   Summary of the video
   In this video, the stone is fairly distal in the duct and stable positioning in the duct is a challenge. One needs to be careful not to be close to the duct wall when using EHL. The tip of the EHL probe is used to stabilise the scope and the stone prior to initiating EHL. Once the stone fragments, the larger fragment is stabilised with the tip of the EHL probe in similar fashion as in the beginning of the video to create fracture points which are progressively expanded with sequential EHL. Maintaining a fluid cushion by irrigation is important, as is reducing the hydrostatic pressure in the ductal system by using suction on the cholangioscope and duodenoscope suction. Energy is still delivered by the EHL probe even when the tip is in direct contact with the stone surface as the cavitation bubble and resultant shock waves are dispersed on either side of the tip of the probe.

3. **Video case 3**

    Title: Stone case 3: EHL

    Summary of the video

    In this video, there is little space or stability around a large stone located low in the bile duct, so the EHL process is carried out by fragmenting an edge of the stone close to the duct wall to enable access to the more central aspect of the stone, from which point, the efficiency of EHL is increased, with stone fragmentation from the centre.

4. **Video case 4**

    Title: Stone case 4: EHL

    Summary of the video

    In this video, the EHL probe is used to progressively cavitate through the stone, facilitating its fragmentation into smaller pieces which can then be individual broken down. Our practice is to maximise the use of EHL during the initial insertion and only remove the cholangioscope to clear fragments once stone fragmentation has been completed or if views are poor and access to more proximal stones needs to be optimised by removing fragments from the distal duct. Successive rounds of EHL may be needed for multiple ductal stones.

5. **Video case 5**

    Title: Stone case 5: EHL

    Summary of the video

    In this video, a cavity has already been created within the stone and the EHL probe is positioned adjacent to the fault line of the cavity to chip off the fragment adjacent to it and optimise fragmentation of the stone.

6. **Video case 6**
   Title: Stone case 6: EHL
   Summary of the video
   In this video, the fracture line created by chipping the surface of the stone is then progressively used to continue EHL and fragmentation with the result that the stone fragments into multiple pieces which can be broken down further. The video additionally demonstrates clear proximal bile ducts once the stone fragments have been extracted.

7. **Video case 7**
   Title: Stone case 7: EHL
   Summary of the video
   In this video, EHL was used to disengage a trapped basket. In the fluoroscopy image, a large stone is seen in the mid-duct with an air-cholangiogram in the proximal duct. Following a biliary sphincterotomy and sphincteroplasty, we attempted stone extraction using an extraction balloon but the size of the stone precluded extraction. A 30 mm Boston Scientific Trapezoid basket was used to engage the stone with a view to crush it and deliver it. However, the basket wires became trapped in the stone during attempts to crush and did not break. The basket wires were cut and the duodenoscope was withdrawn. Attempts to insert the emergency lithotripter sheath over the wires of the basket were unsuccessful as these wires were not as stiff as the wires of a mechanical lithotripter. The duodenoscope was reinserted and a SpyGlass cholangioscope was inserted into the bile duct adjacent to the trapped basket wires. EHL was performed on the stone and following stone fragmentation, the basket wires were released and removed. EHL was continued until the stone was completely fragmented and an extraction balloon was used to clear

stone fragments from the duct with complete duct clearance.

Strictures

1. **Video case 8**
   Title: Stricture 1
   Summary of the video
   This video illustrates the cholangioscopic appearance of an advanced cholangiocarcinoma occupying the common hepatic duct and the liver hilum. This is a Bismuth Type IV tumour extending from the hilum where the cholangioscope is positioned, into the right and left intraductal systems. The cholangioscope is inserted into the right posterior sectoral system where the second order ducts are noted to be uninvolved. The cholangioscope is withdrawn over a guidewire after biopsies are acquired from the mass in the hilar area.

2. **Video case 9**
   Title: Stricture 2
   Summary of the video
   In this video, an advanced, stricturing tumour is seen extending from the common hepatic duct into the left and right intraductal systems which are selectively cannulated using the cholangioscope. Biopsies from the tumour revealed cholangiocarcinoma.

3. **Video case 10**
   Title: Indeterminate biliary stricture: tissue ingrowth into SEMS
   Summary of the video
   In this video, cholangioscopy was performed for tissue acquisition in a patient who had had a previous partially covered biliary self-expanding metal stent (SEMS)

inserted across a distal bile duct stricture which was presumed to be malignant, but brush cytology was negative. The video demonstrates the use of the Spybite forceps which is inserted through the meshwork of the stent in order to acquire tissue off the duct wall.

Other

1. **Video case 11**
   Title: Stone concretions around a coil
   Summary of the video
   A patient underwent embolization of a branch of a bleeding gastroduodenal artery from a duodenal ulcer many years ago and presented with recurrent cholangitis. Cross-sectional imaging revealed that the coil had migrated into the bile duct and had developed a stone around it. Cholangioscopy demonstrated large concretions around the coil, which were fragmented using EHL, enabling release of the coil, which was delivered from the bile duct using a basket.

2. **Video case 12**
   Title: Pancreatoscopy and EHL
   Summary of the video
   This video demonstrates the technique of pancreatoscopy and EHL for treating large pancreatic stones. This patient with chronic pancreatitis presented with symptoms of obstructive pancreatopathy (post prandial pancreatic pain and worsening pancreatic exocrine insufficiency). A large stone was seen in the main pancreatic duct in the head of the pancreas with a dilated main duct proximal to the stone. Access to the stone was achieved with a combination of pancreatic sphincterotomy and dilatation of a main duct stricture distal

to the stone. Unlike in the bile duct, manoeuvrability within the pancreatic duct is limited and care must be taken during irrigation within the main duct. EHL was performed sequentially and stone fragments are subsequently cleared using small baskets.

Video B: Spyglass Cholangioscopy Video Transcript

Introduction and Set Up

Dr. Richard Sturgess
"Single operator cholangioscopy is a relatively new technique now with a digital platform that's used in conjunction with ERCP to deal with advanced biliary disease, particularly complex stones and indeterminate strictures.

With this short video what we want to illustrate is some of the practical aspects of setting up the Boston Scientific Spyglass Digital Cholangioscope together with some tips and tricks for its use.

So, Emma, do you want to start setting up the kit as we normally would."

Emma Langley

"Spyglass: most importantly, what we would always check is the expiry date. Now the expiry date can be found here on the box and it can also be found here as well. So before opening the kit always check your expiry dates."

Dr. Richard Sturgess

"Emma, it's a single pack with everything in it that's required for the actual cholangioscopy".

Emma Langley

"This is how the packet arrives and this just contains the DS Spyscope, nothing else. We would take the camera out of the package and the first thing that I do take it over to here to connect. So, then I unravel it… so, this is just removing the protective sheath that it was packaged in…then we are going to look to these two pieces here, we can attach suction here, we can also attach saline from an irrigation pump to here. This irrigation tubing… goes firstly into a bottle of saline here, and we do have a little screw on the cap to make sure that's tight, it then connects to this bit of kit here. These two markers here indicate where the tubing needs to sit in the actual pump itself… and close the lid on the pump. Always ensure that it is turned on. Then we connect to this part of the DS … it's got the water-mark here."

Dr. Richard Sturgess

"So we've got suction there and irrigation there and that's it ready to use isn't it?"

Emma Langley

"The Spyglass is ready to use now yes; you can actually use the foot pedal to check the pump to ensure that the saline is flushing through."

Dr. Richard Sturgess
"Okay, we'll talk a bit more about the kit in a second, but we've taken a time over that, but you can normally set a DS Spyglass up ready to go in under a minute, can't you?"

Emma Langley
"Yes, you can, it's just all about getting use to the kit."

Dr. Richard Sturgess
"And just checking the sell by dates".

Emma Langley
"Checking the use by dates on everything, or your expiries and then the more you do it the more natural it becomes."

Dr. Richard Sturgess
"Making sure it's the right direction in the pump as well so it pumps out not in. Okay that's about it.

I think what we should do now is have look at some of the components of the actual hardware that sells."

Hardware Used

Dr. Richard Sturgess
"So, what I'm going to do now is just go through some of the actual bits of hardware that you will need to undertake Spyglass cholangioscopy.

Clearly this is an ERCP technique so your duodenoscope and its associated bits and bobs to allow us to do ERCP but when you look specifically at the cholangioscopy aspects of the procedure, the critical bit of kit is the actual Spyglass DS visualisation system here. We saw earlier how the disposable part plugs in, it's a small piece of kit that will fit very easily on a standard trolley, on and off switches there; the light can go on and off with this button there and you can manually adjust the light. It really couldn't be much simpler than that in terms of using the Spyglass kit, it really is plug and play. Out it comes, in it goes, ready to use, light comes on.

We talked about the pump, that irrigation is tremendously important with cholangioscopy, there is a lot of muck and goo in the bile duct and the ability to irrigate and aspirate at the same time and clean up the bile duct is one of the key features that allows effective single operator cholangioscopy.

And the other bit of hardware that is frequently used is some form of energy generator to do lithotripsy, so that can be electro-hydronic or laser. In this situation, we've got here Autolith Electro Hydraulic Lithotriptor, again very simple to use. It's got a foot pedal down here that just feeds in: it's an air pressure standard activated foot pedal. You can see it's waiting for us to connect the probe just here and we can adjust the power level both in number of pulses, so I can increase that fairly steadily from one to thirty and then down again. We normally start on fifteen shots and then the power has got three settings, low medium and high. We normally start on medium but fairly rapidly if need be move on to high power.

And that's about it really for the hardware that's required for cholangioscopy: two solid bits of kit for actually driving it and the pump for irrigating."

Monitoring

Dr. Richard Sturgess

"When one is undertaking cholangioscopy there is clearly a lot of visual image input.

This is how we set up our screen, we have a Spy image that you can see on the left, we have an endoscopy image top centre, we obviously have live and reference fluoro that occurs in the other blank screens; clearly we haven't got a patient and they are not irradiating here, so cholangioscopy, endoscopy, live and reference fluoro and in a non-anaesthetised case, the patients vitals as we see here. And manipulation of this screen allows you to optimise the views so a lot of the time when one is undertaking the cholangioscopy you don't need the bigger screen for duodenoscopy and you concentrate on the cholangioscopy with your other main screen being fluoroscopy, but the ability to change round and have these multiple inputs easily accessible within everyone's visual field is clearly very advantageous when undertaking complex procedures like cholangioscopy."

Practical Aspects of Using the Equipment

Dr. Richard Sturgess

"So now we're going to illustrate some of the practical aspects of using the Spyglass cholangioscope with a duodenoscope and how we actually insert it. Clearly, we haven't got a patient here so there will be some slightly artificial elements to this, but it should be able to illustrate the points. One of the things you'll notice is that we've got a second nurse here, Laura, and it's a good point to make, as this is a complex procedure and you certainly need two assistants working the wires, as well as another assistant helping out with the patient and being generally a third pair of hands around; there is a lot to do here and you do need the hands.

Right, so let's put the Cholangioscope up, and instantly the first thing we can see is that it is quite difficult with the light so, when actually putting this on the wire it's better to turn the light off and then it's much easier for the nursing assistant to actually place it over the wire.

So, the majority of the times you are using the Cholangioscope you are probably going to want to do a standard wire guided approach… slide it over and your wire is in the bile duct, but it is possible to cannulate free hand particularly through a mature sphincterotomy and sometimes with a very wide duct when you know you are going to be straight away into dealing with stones, I won't put it over a wire, I'll preload a lithotriptor and do a free-hand cannulation.

So, if Laura holds the scope here as it was in the patient, so we've got a short-wire system here, Boston short-wire, so I'm going to un-clip that and then as standard… very easy… slides in… nice and easily… down the scope… down it goes… quite happily. So we're using this with a short-wire system, a 260 wire and we've got enough length with the 260 to get out and get control on both sides of the wire and gripping the other end with a bridge as you normally would so you do not need long wire systems to do this. And I'm just down at the bridge now and out is the cholangioscope coming as we can see just here. So that is effectively the cholangioscope in the duodenum, now at this stage what I normally do is put the handle on so I will un-clip my short wire device and then Emma is going to put the handle in place, so we are just going to use our hands together, you've got to start to learn to work this, there is the rubber strap that comes across… always a bit of an effort to get on but it does hold it very securely, so that's quite a long rubber strap. Let's just illustrate that, so here you've got the handle which I'll go through in a bit more detail in a second, the handle is sitting here, it's held on with this, robust, and you just saw how robust it is to get on, this robust rubber strap and that holds it quite

Video B: Spyglass Cholangioscopy Video Transcript

firmly, there's a bit of rotational movement possible but it is actually firm enough to use.

So, what I would normally do at this stage now is to cannulate the bile duct with a little bit of tension on the wire and we go up like that and into where we want to go.

So, let's look at the handle now and you'll see the parallel, I'll just hold this in a slightly un-natural way from when it was in a patient, we've got the standard duodenoscope and these are replicated on the SpyScope, up and down, left and right. And very usefully there is a brake on there that will hold it in a position but still allow you to move it.

So looking at the cholangioscope now, we've got up and down movement in both directions, and we've also got left and right, not quite as precise as you'll get with an endoscope but this is really very good movement which will allow you to get deeply into the intrahepatic ducts with good vision and the ability to look around and this is a real advance this four way movement and we can put the locks on.

Okay, so if we come back to the actual duodenoscope handle itself and how I use my hands.

My left hand is doing the conventional control of the duodenoscope as you would normally, and my right hand is sitting here using the cholangioscope controls. I almost always have the brake on to stabilise the tip of the cholangioscope when I'm manoeuvring the cholangioscope within the biliary and sometimes the pancreatic duct.

Let's look at what we've actually got in addition to the control wheels. We've also got our accessory channel which is currently got the wire in which we will move in a second and then go through putting an accessory down, but also usefully here we have our suction which we can turn on and off. If we want to do a cholangiogram, we can either inject down the biopsy accessory channel or the irrigation channel as required. But if you are doing that you do need to turn the suction off, otherwise the contrast medium will just be sucked up instantly. So, it's got an on off control… Emma why don't you just take the pump off and we'll just illustrate the pump.

Okay let's just illustrate the pump, this is quite a vigorous pump I'll just hold it here, if you can focus in there that will be great… so the pump that we've got here is quite powerful you can see it jetting out fluid there. That is great in some respects in that it allows us to irrigate very effectively in the bile duct but you do have to be careful if you are upstream of a stricture; you could inject a lot of washing fluid, saline, quite quickly and under pressure and it is something to be very cautious with when you are upstream of a stricture; and one of the few excess complications that we see with cholangioscopy over and above ERCP, is infection and that's the particular situation when you can have a high pressure jet going above a stricture and potentially causing translocation of bacteria that way.

Okay, let's look at the accessories now that we have put down. Say we are going biopsy a stricture we would take the wire out, we've got deep access here… and then we are going to take a biopsy forceps… again they come in the standard box… (the expiry dates are here) so these are the Spybite forceps, they are 1.2 mm in diameter, about 280 cm in length… Do you want to see if you can get really tight on this and we can just have a look at this? So, we can see the biopsy forceps open there, and shut, okay, really fine. The other practical point is that the tip of the biopsy forceps is not very flexible. Further on down, very flexible but that first perhaps 3 or 4 cm is not terribly flexible and that sometimes causes a bit of an issue getting the biopsy forceps out of the cholangioscope. With the new digital cholangioscope it is undoubtably easier than it was previously. So, these, as you would imagine,

Video B: Spyglass Cholangioscopy Video Transcript

very straight forwardly go straight down the biopsy channel, very very easy… down it goes… right, if we can go back to the cholangioscope tip now, so the biopsy forceps exit out into direct vision and operating them is absolutely the same as operating any other biopsy forceps, you press up against the lesion that you want to biopsy, close down and away you come, it's as straight forward as that and everything that you would imagine. We normally aim to take four, five or six biopsies, it can be quite difficult getting the biopsy forceps out of the end of the cholangioscope but once they've been out once you usually find the biopsy forceps pass relatively easily. It can be a little bit time consuming to take these number of biopsy's but there's no doubt that if you do get to six biopsy's or more, you're going to increase your yield of accurate histological diagnosis.

The only other regular piece of kit that we use is a electrohydraulic lithotripsy (EHL) fibre… (**Emma Langley**: expiry dates are here) … so here's the Autolith; we'll need a power lead Emma, again very similar, passes down the access channel very easily… so down it comes… last little bit comes out… and the Autolith probe comes out, we connect to the power lead so that is now connected to the energy generator and we've got the foot pedal down here to deliver the pulses. So with the EHL probe we won't have an aiming beam we can just clearly see it in there, if you're using a laser lithotripsy device there is normally an aiming beam that is activated so you can see the direction of the energy that you release when firing.

So, those are the two common use accessories, there is also now available; two other accessories which we won't open out but discuss… So, here we have the Boston Scientific Spyglass Retrieval Snare, it's not an electrosurgical snare it's a mechanical device, there is the potential for harvesting tissue with it but it's main use is object removal and in particular migrated stent retrieval, and the other device is the Boston Scientific Retrieval Basket and this is aimed at the stone work particularly for difficult small intrahepatic stones but also migrated objects including stents.

When you're doing particularly stone disease, it may be that you are removing the Spyglass cholangioscope two or three times during a procedure to subsequently remove stones and then go back in and do more lithotripsy, take it out; as I say with a mature sphincterotomy this can be very quick, you can freehand cannulate. If you are passing over the wire each time, it's again pretty quick and there is a standard wire exchange. This is the digital version of the SpyScope now in its second iteration, it is undoubtably considerably easier to use than the legacy SpyScope with its fibre optic configuration.

So, I think that is about everything that we need to say about the Spyglass it is straight forward to use in principle, there's a lot of skills to be learnt both for the nursing staff and the ERC operator/ERCP'ist.

Thank you very much."

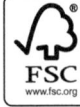

MIX
Papier aus verantwortungsvollen Quellen
Paper from responsible sources
FSC® C105338

If you have any concerns about our products,
you can contact us on
ProductSafety@springernature.com

In case Publisher is established outside the EU,
the EU authorized representative is:
**Springer Nature Customer Service Center GmbH
Europaplatz 3, 69115 Heidelberg, Germany**

Printed by Libri Plureos GmbH
in Hamburg, Germany